5 Steps to
A Healthy and Safe Pregnancy

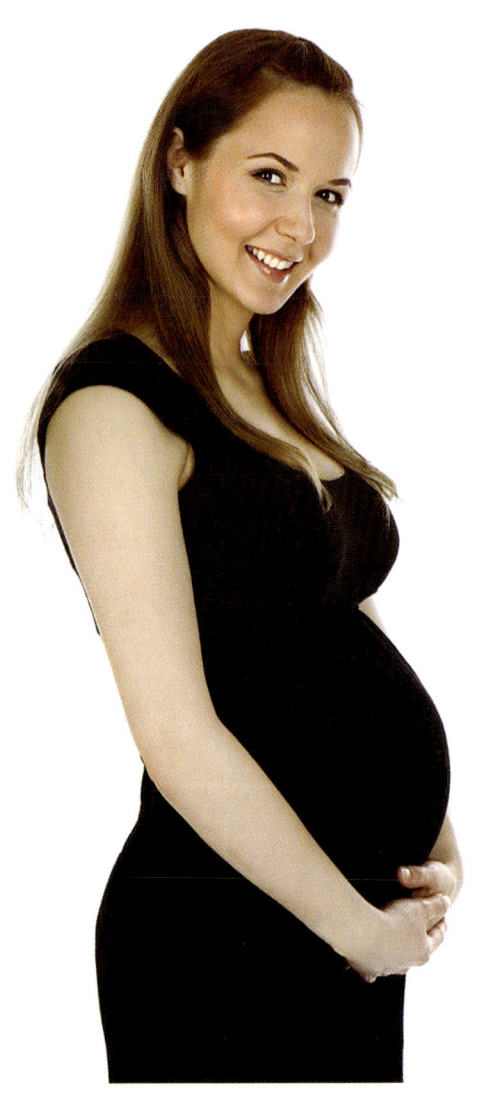

Learn about

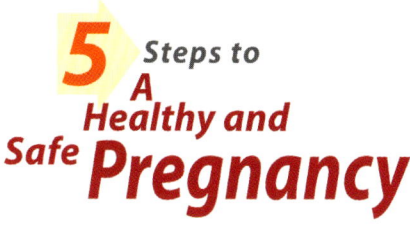

5 Steps to A Healthy and Safe Pregnancy

Dr. ANJALI ARORA
DR. VRINDA ARORA

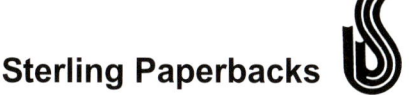

STERLING PAPERBACKS
An imprint of
Sterling Publishers (P) Ltd.
A-59, Okhla Industrial Area, Phase-II,
New Delhi-110020.
Tel: 26387070, 26386209; Fax: 91-11-26383788
E-mail: mail@sterlingpublishers.com
ghai@nde.vsnl.net.in
www.sterlingpublishers.com

5 Steps to
A Healthy and Safe Pregnancy
© 2011, *Dr. Anjali Arora & Dr. Vrinda Arora*
ISBN 978 81 207 4922 1

The author wishes to thank all academicians, scientists and writers who have been a source of inspiration.

The author and publisher specifically disclaim any liability, loss or risk, whatsoever, personal or otherwise, which is incurred as a consequence, directly or indirectly of the use and application of any of the contents of this book.

All rights are reserved.
No part of this publication may be reproduced, stored in a retrieval system or transmitted, in any form or by any means, mechanical, photocopying, recording or otherwise, without prior written permission of the authors.

Printed and Published by Sterling Publishers Pvt. Ltd., New Delhi-110020.

Contents

1. Preparation for Motherhood — 8
2. Trimesters of Pregnancy — 25
3. Diseases Affecting Mother and Foetus — 34
4. Healthy Eating with Safe Exercise During Pregnancy — 58
5. Later Half of Pregnancy and the "D Day" — 73

   Myths and Fact File — 80

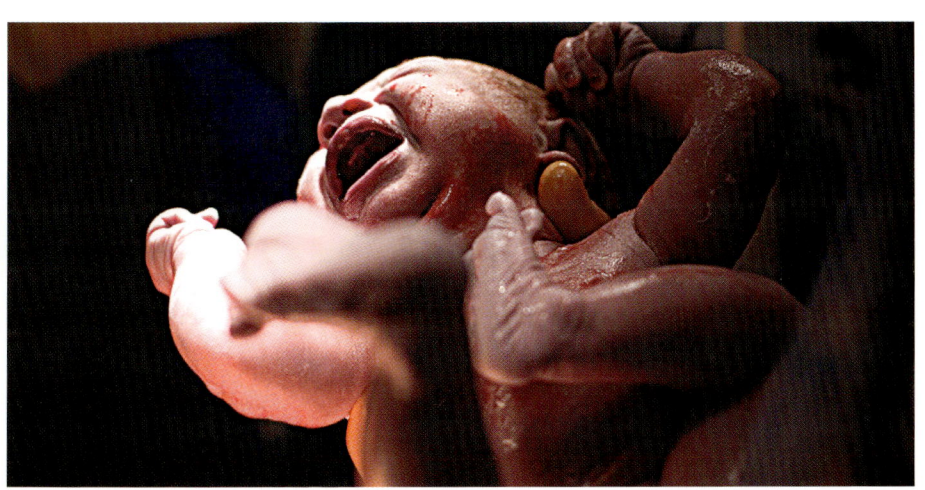

Are you aware of some of these factors?

1. **A woman conceives when**
   a) An ovum fuses with another ovum
   b) An ovum fuses with a sperm
   c) An ovum fuses with the tube
2. **Pregnancy can be detected by a blood test**
   a) After 45 days of conception
   b) After 30 days of conception
   c) After 15 days of conception
3. **Fertility in a woman starts diminishing around**
   a) 40 yrs of age
   b) 30 yrs of age
   c) 20 yrs of age
4. **To avoid sagging of muscles after delivery, it is important to start exercising around**
   a) First week of delivery
   b) 40 days after delivery
   c) 6 months after delivery

The above questionnaire will help you find out as to how aware you are of pregnancy. If you answer more of (b), then you are aware about a healthy pregnancy.

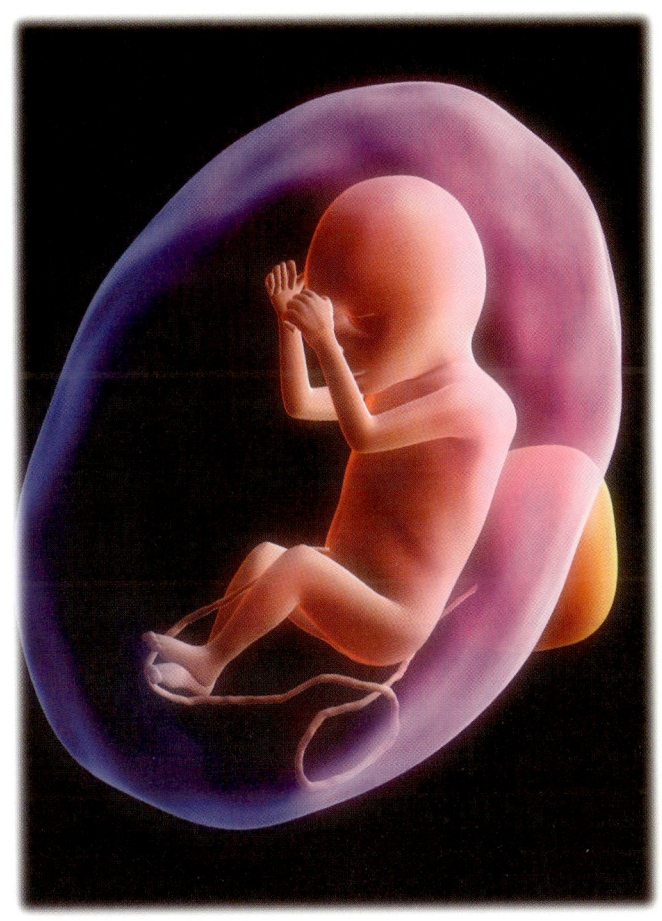

Preparation for Motherhood

Marriage and Pregnancy

Teen marriages or pregnancies are common in the Western world like their counterparts of "child marriage" in the East. Child marriage is defined as any marriage carried out below 18 years of age. The girl at this stage, is not ready physically, physiologically or psychologically to fulfill the responsibilities of marriage and childbearing. Child marriage is related to multiple health risks. Also pregnancy related deaths are high in girls between 15-19 years of age.

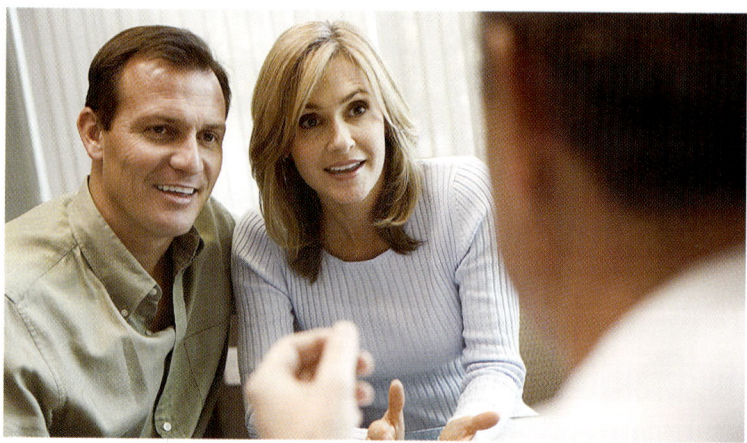

Divorce rate among couples under twenty years is known to be high (between 80-85%). Social scientists have found that people who marry young are seldom prepared for marital roles.

On the other hand, there is a gradual decrease in fertility among women after the age of 30. As the age progresses a woman may take longer to conceive, or she may have to face the problems of sub-fertility or infertility.

Women starting a family in their late 20s or early 30s might lead a healthier lifestyle. They are often more educated and better off financially. They may understand the needs of their bodies and look after themselves better in terms of exercise and nutrition. Mature women have more positive perceptions of their bodies, and more readily tolerate the symptoms of pregnancy. At this age women are often independent, confident and know what they want.

It is also a well known fact that older women (>35 years) have a higher chance of having a baby with a genetic abnormality, such as Down's syndrome. There is a marked pattern of increased intervention with the

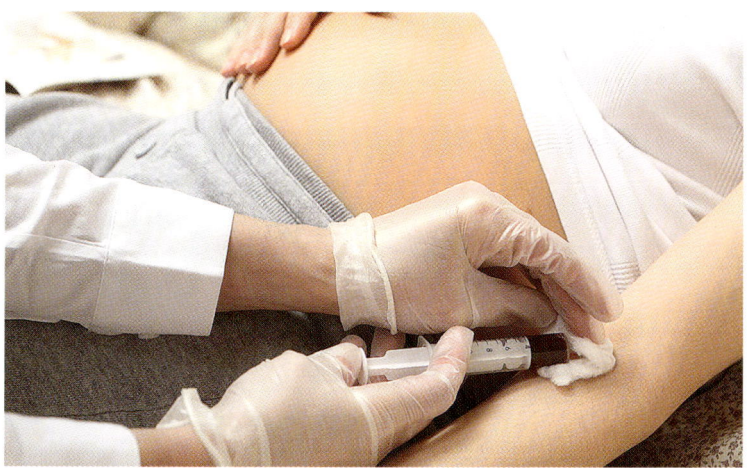

increasing age of the mother. Virtually all studies agree that the rate of caesareans also rise with maternal age.

Once you are prepared for pregnancy and you have decided to go for it, get a general checkup done, to detect if you are suffering from any of the following :-

- Anaemia
- Thyroid disease
- Diabetes mellitus
- High blood pressure
- Thalassaemia

or any other disease which may affect your pregnancy.

Also check if you have been vaccinated with Rubella vaccine.

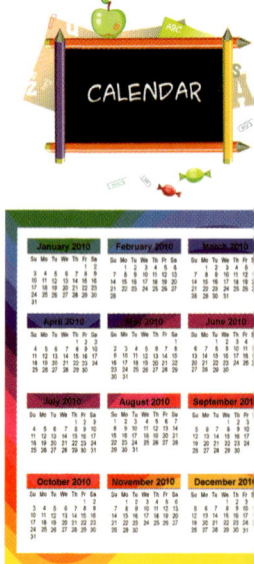

Pregnancy and Conception

Every woman must have an idea of the anatomy of her reproductive system. She also must note the date of her menstrual cycle in a diary or calender. Before marriage the young lady must be aware of her ovulation time, i.e. the most fertile period. Calculation of pregnancy is from the first day of the last menstrual period.

Ovulation –

Every month, in the woman's ovaries, a group of immature eggs start to develop in small fluid-filled cysts called follicles. Normally, one of the follicles is selected to complete development (maturation). This is called the 'dominant follicle'. The dominant follicle ruptures and releases the egg from the ovary (ovulation). Ovulation generally occurs about two weeks or (14 days) before a woman's next menstrual period begins (i.e. mid-cycle).

Preparation of the Corpus Luteum –

After ovulation, the ruptured follicle develops into a structure called the corpus luteum, which secretes two hormones – progesterone and estrogen. Progesterone helps prepare the endometrium (lining of the uterus) for the embryo to be implanted.

Fate of the Egg (ovum) –

The egg travels into the fallopian tube where it remains until a single sperm penetrates it during fertilization. The egg can be fertilized for about 24 hours after ovulation.

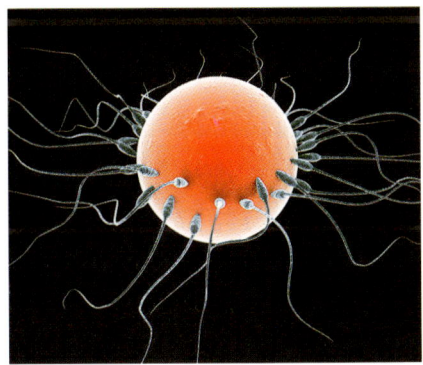

Menstruation –

If no sperm fertilises the egg, the corpus luteum degenerates, reducing or decreasing (ovum) the levels of hormones. This causes the endometrium to slough off, leading to menstruation. This is often known as "weeping of the uterus" as no fertilization took place.

Fertilization –

When the sperm penetrates the egg (ovum), changes occur in the protein coating around the egg (ovum) to prevent other sperms from entering. On fertilization, the baby's genetic make-up is complete, including its sex. The mother can provide only XX chromosomes. The father provides the XY chromosomes. If a Y sperm (from the father) fertilizes the egg, the baby will be a boy (XY) and if an X sperm from the father fertilizes the egg, the baby will be a girl (XX).

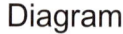

Diagram

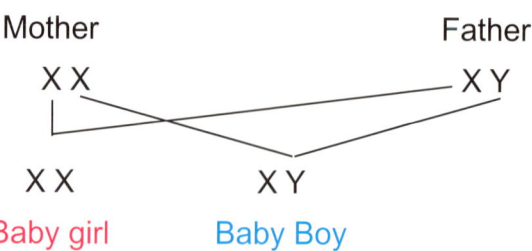

Implantation –

The fertilized egg undergoes a number of changes before implanting itself on to the endometrium. The endometrium at this stage, becomes thicker and the cervix gets sealed by a mucus plug. The gradually developing cells form the "embryo". The "embryo stage" is defined from the moment of conception to the eighth week of pregnancy. After the eighth week until the baby is born the developing baby is known as "the foetus".

Symptoms of Pregnancy

The first symptom of pregnancy is normally the absence of the menstrual period in a woman. Other symptoms that may indicate pregnancy are:

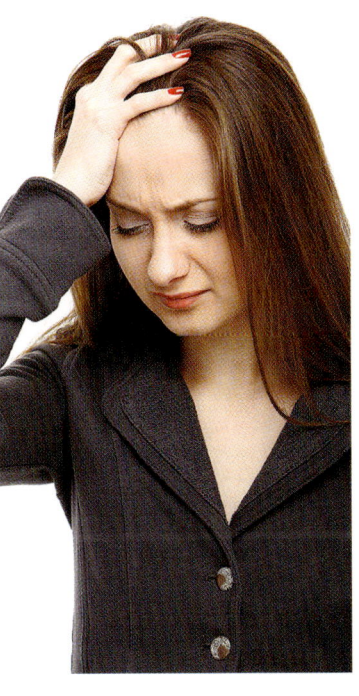

- Fatigue
- Morning sickness
- Tenderness and swelling in the breasts
- Frequent urination
- Cravings for certain food items like sweets and rich carbohydrate foods (chocolates, pastries, pizza, pies, kulfi, *channa bhatura*)
- Backache

Pregnancy tests

- Home pregnancy tests: These kit tests are available at your chemist shop. Principle of the test assay is to detect raised levels of the hormone HCG (human chorionic gonadotropin) in the urine. Before using your kit read the instructions given.
- The pregnancy test if positive must be followed by a visit to your obstetrician.

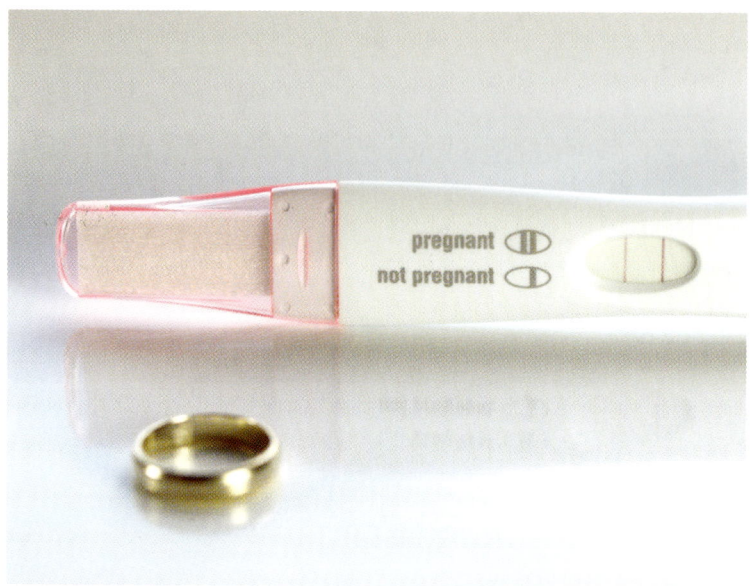

To Calculate EDD (Estimated Delivery Date)

A pregnancy normally remains till 280 days or 9 months and 7 days or 40 weeks, i.e. if a woman's last period was on 25th June then counting 9 months, it calculates to 25th March. Adding 7 days, the EDD would be 1st April.

Initial Examination/Routine Tests Conducted During First Trimester of Pregnancy:-

- Height / Weight
- Blood pressure
- Urine test, for albumin and sugar
- Blood group with Rh
- Blood Sugar (Fasting and Post Parandial)
- Complete Blood count

- Thyroid Function Test
- Blood tests for HIV, Hepatitis B, Rubella, VDRL (Venereal Disease Research Laboratory)
- Ultrasound
- HPLC is done for Thalassaemic screening

Specialised tests required for First trimester screening.

Blood Test:-

- Maternal Serum Alpha Fetoprotein (MSAFP)
- Pregnancy associated placental protein - A (PAPP-A)
- HcG

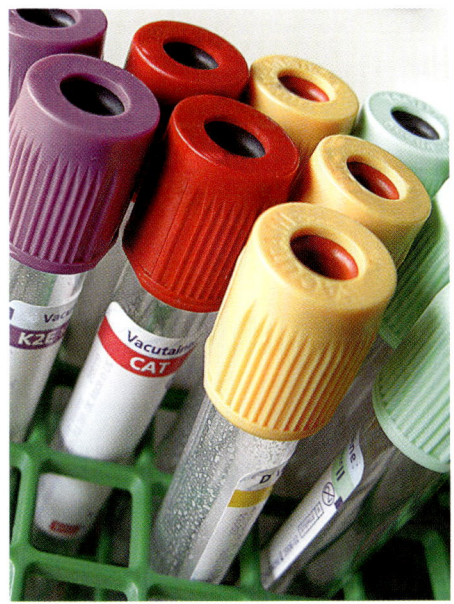

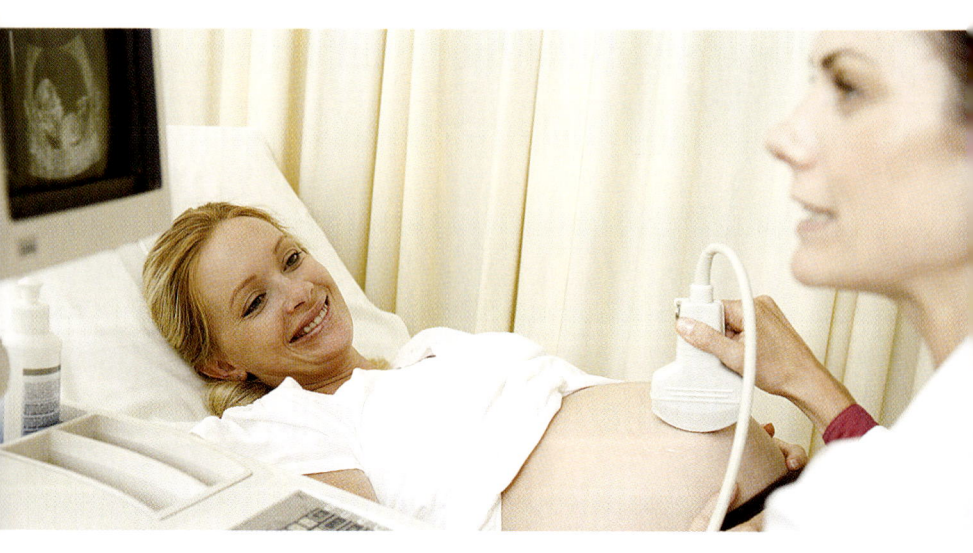

Ultrasound for:-

- Nuchal translucency (NT)
- Nasal bone (NB)

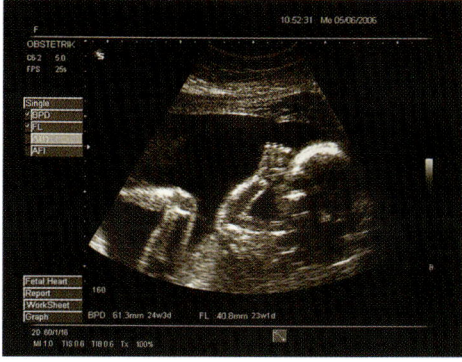

You must go for the ultrasound with a full bladder. You will be asked to lie down on the bed next to the ultrasound machine. A gel will be spread over the abdomen. Then, a small device (like a computer mouse) is slowly moved over your abdomen and the doctor studies the scan on the machine screen. Photographs of the foetus are also taken and kept for future comparison.

Rh blood group

The card stating your blood group and Rh factor (positive or negative) should always be carried in your purse. If you are Rh negative and your husband is Rh positive, the chances are that your baby may also be Rh positive. During the birth of the baby, the baby's blood may leak into your blood circulation. Your body will then respond to the baby's blood (if it is Rh+ve) by producing antibodies against the Rh factor. This can cause jaundice and anaemia in the next baby (if the baby is Rh+ve). To avoid this, injection of Anti D immunoglobin is given to the Rh negative mother, at twenty-eight weeks of gestation and then within 72 hours after the birth of the Rh + ve baby. After each delivery, abortion or miscarriage, the Rh negative mother should receive an injection of Anti Dimmunoglobin.

Tests Conducted During Second Trimester of Pregnancy

- **Routine Screening for the mother**

Checking of Weight

Blood pressure recording

Testing urine for albumin and sugar

For any anomalies Ultrasound Anomaly Scan (18-20 weeks)

- **Maternal serum screening test**

This test is usually taken between 15 to 20 weeks of pregnancy. It checks for birth defects such as Down's syndrome, open neural tube defect, etc. It is also known as a Triple screen test.

If your routine screening tests are positive for congenital anomalies then Diagnostic tests like the following are conducted:

- Amniocentesis
- Chronic Villus Sampling (CVS)
- Chordocentesis

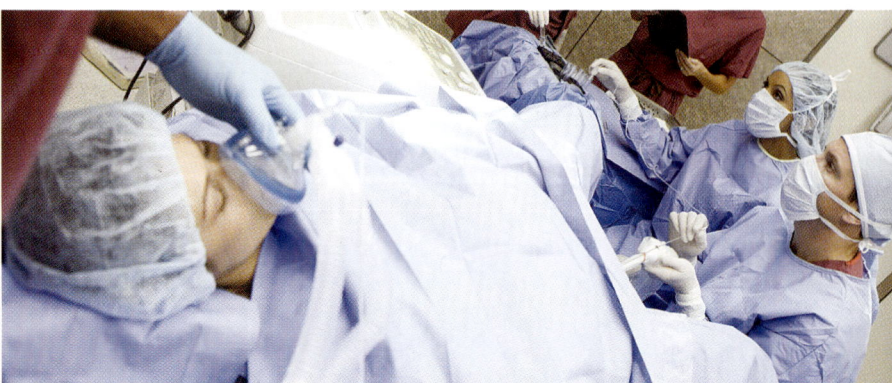

Glucose screening test –

Irrespective of what meal you have had, 50 gms of oral glucose is given to you and a blood sugar test is conducted after an hour.

– Glucose challange Test (screening test) is conducted between 26-28 weeks of pregnancy. Level of blood sugar should be less than 140mg /dl.

This helps to screen gestational diabetes, a form of diabetes that develops in the mother during pregnancy.

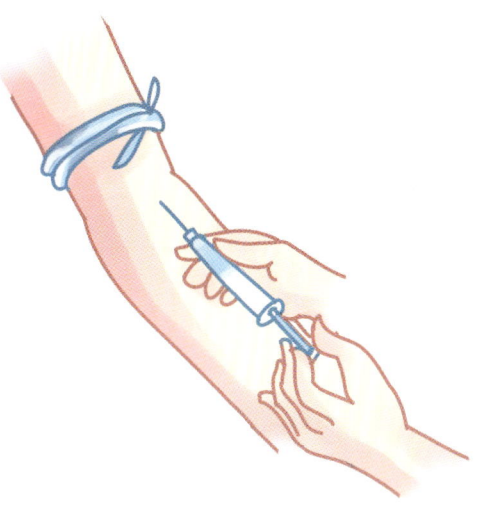

Tests Conducted During Third Trimester of Pregnancy

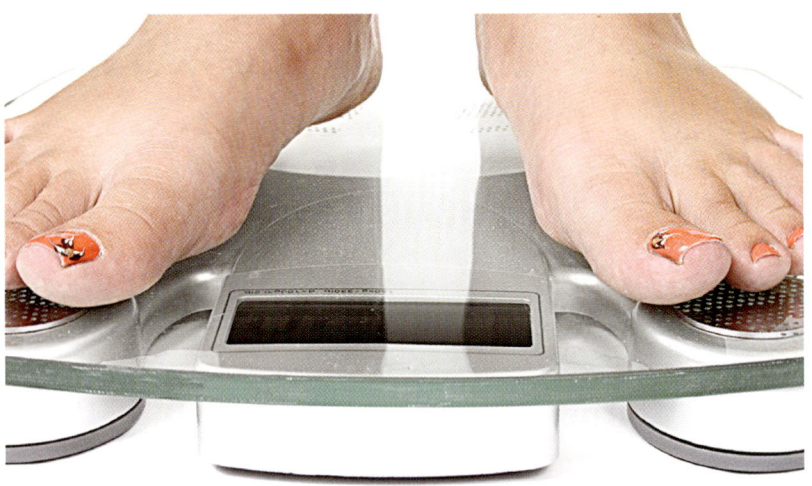

Routine Examination
Checking of Weight
Blood pressure recording

Testing urine
First morning sample of urine is preferable.

Urine (routine and microscopic).

Diseases to be detected during pregnancy:

- **Placenta praevia**

The placenta abnormally lies in the lower section of the uterus. This completely or partially covers the cervix hindering a vaginal delivery.

- **Down's syndrome**

It is a genetic disorder in which an individual has an extra 21st chromosome resulting in mental retardation, heart and kidney disease.

- **Neural Tube defects**

e.g. spina bifida

- **Cystic fibrosis**
- **Tay Sachs Disease**
- **Other diseases like tumours, congenital heart disease, etc.**

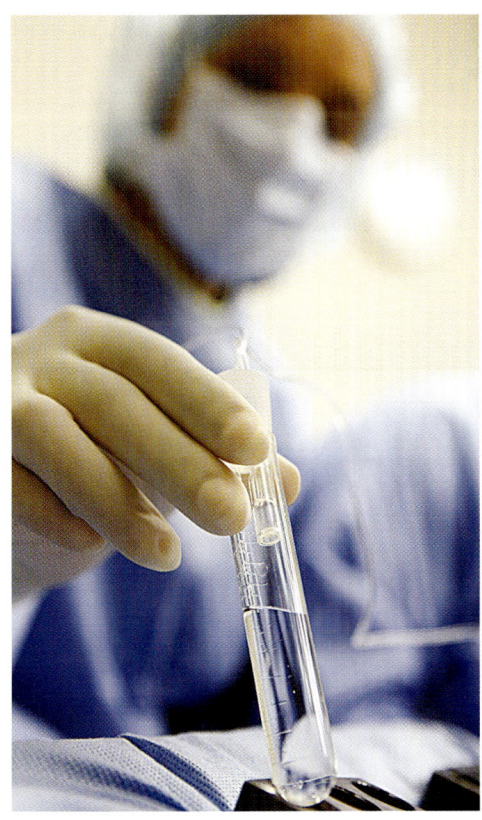

Infertility

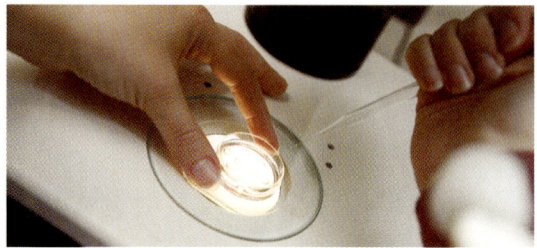

IVF or In Vitro Fertilization

Conception normally occurs by the fusion of sperm (male sex cell) and egg (female sex cell), inside the woman's womb. IVF or In Vitro Fertilization is the fertilization of a female egg with a male's sperm outside the body under special conditions. In IVF, the sperms and eggs are fused (fertilized), in special tubes and petridishes in the IVF laboratory. Special incubators are used to keep these sperms and eggs together in an environment similar to the mother's womb. On successful fertilization, these embryos (earliest form of the baby) are transferred into the mother's uterus. This procedure is known as Embryo Transfer or ET.

Causes of infertility in the mother

- Unknown
- Absent tubes or damaged fallopian tubes
- Tuberculosis
- Endometriosis
- Antibodies against sperms in the cervix
- Poor or no egg formation by the ovaries

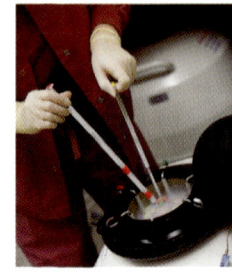

Causes of infertility in the father
- Abnormal sperm count
- Presence of defective sperms
- Decrease in sperum motility

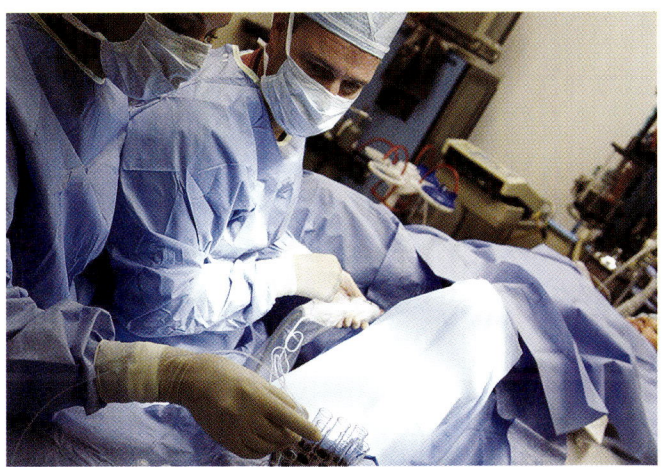

IVF Procedure

IVF does not involve any surgical procedure. It does not require a cut or stitch. For the procedure, the ovaries are stimulated on the 2nd day of the menstrual cycle with the help of certain medication. After stimulation, the follicles present in the ovaries take 12-14 days to develop fully. It is at this stage that eggs are aspirated out from the ovaries. The egg collection is done under sedation or a short general anaesthesia. A needle is inserted through the vagina and under ultrasound guidance, the eggs are collected from both the ovaries. This procedure normally takes 15-30 minutes. Soon after the eggs are obtained, the partner is asked to collect a semen sample by masturbation.

Embryo Transfer

After fertilisation takes place embryos are transferred after two to three days. Embryos are transferred into the uterine cavity through the vagina with the help of special fine catheters. ET is a painless procedure and no anaesthesia is required. Normally 3-4 embryos are transferred if ET is done on the second or third day. However, if ET is done on the fourth or fifth day at an advanced stage of embryo development, only 1 to 2 embryos are sufficient to cause a successful pregnancy. (Every country has their own rules for embryo transfer).

Complications of IVF

The drugs used for stimulating egg development in ovaries can sometimes excessively stimulate ovaries leading to a symptom complex known as Ovarian Hyper-Stimulation Syndrome (OHSS). Multiple pregnancy is another risk which can occur in a patient undergoing IVF.

Women who can opt for IVF

- Those under the age of 35 trying to conceive for more than a year. (with unexplained infertility)
- Those over the age of 35 who have been trying to conceive for six months
- Having blocked or damaged fallopian tubes
- Having ovulation disorders
- Sufferring from Severe Endometeriosis (damaging the tubes)
- Low sperm count (in partner)
- Sperm immotility (in partner)

2   *Trimesters of Pregnancy*

First Trimester

The first month: After conception the baby for the first 8 to 9 weeks is called an embryo. In the first month embryonic development of the heart, lungs and brain starts. The heart starts beating around the 25th day of conception. The embryo is enclosed in a sac of fluid and grows in this sac until birth. This sac of fluid helps protect the embryo from injury. The umbilical cord connecting the embryo and the mother supplies blood and nourishment to the embryo. At this stage, the pregnant woman starts feeling tenderness in her breast. Some mothers also develop 'morning sickness' or nausea.

The second month:

The embryo becomes a foetus after 13-28 weeks. It has arms with tiny hands and fingers. Legs show the early development of knees, ankles, and toes. Organs such as the stomach, liver, brain, spine and central nervous system also start developing. Pits become the baby's eyes and ears. The mother at this stand may get tired more easily. She may need to urinate more frequently. Some nausea may be present. Therefore, proper nourishment must be kept in mind.

The third month: By the end of this trimester, the signs of the foetus's sex begins. Facial features become well defined, e.g. development of chin, nose, and forehead. The foetus starts to move hands, legs, and head. At this point the foetus's movement is not felt. Testing of urine, blood pressure and weight should be recorded on each visit to the doctor.

Second Trimester

The fourth month: By the end of this month, the foetus is now about 8 to 10 inches long. The mother now looks prominent with her weight gain.

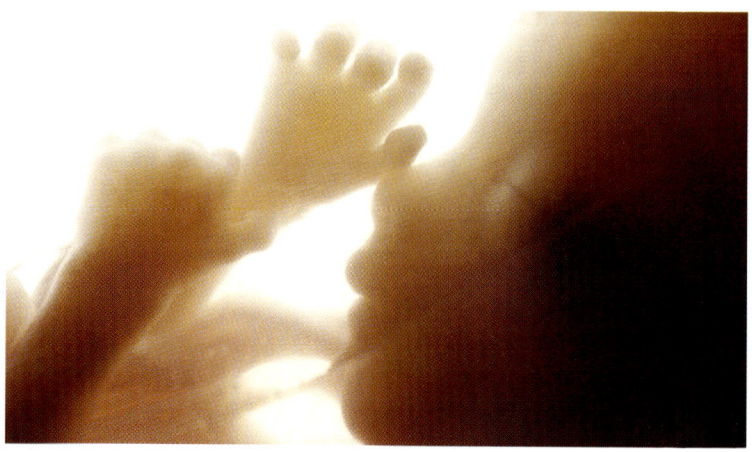

The fifth month: At this stage, the doctor can hear the foetus's heartbeat. The movements of the foetus get stronger and are felt at about 18-20 weeks of pregnancy. If there is no movement by the beginning of the fifth month, the doctor should be consulted. Eyes, eyelids and ears of the foetus are now fully developed. Fine hair, known as lanugo covers the baby's body. Visits to the doctor should be every four weeks during this trimester. During the visit the baby's heartbeat is heard. The foetus's development and age are determined through ultrasound. Urine and blood pressure are seen on every visit.

The sixth month: A fully formed foetus is now in the mother's womb. The foetus's skin is wrinkled and red and there is practically no fat under the skin. The growing foetus is now is about 14 inches long. The eyelids of the foetus open. The number of brain tissues start increasing at this stage.

Symptoms which can occur

- Swelling of the hands and feet which should be relieved on rest,
- Quickening is perceptions of foetal movements

As the pregnancy progresses, everyday activities such as sitting and standing can become uncomfortable. The mother should try and move around every couple of hours. This helps prevent fluid buildup in the legs and feet. At the same time it eases muscle tension.

Also try the following:

- **Sitting -** A firm seat and back cushions to be used. This gives support to the lower back and can make for long hours of sitting much easier. Put the feet up on a foot rest or a waste basket in the office or home.
- **Standing -** Prolonged standing can cause blood to pool in the legs. This can lead to pain or dizziness. Wear comfortable shoes and if one must stand for long periods of time, put one of your feet up on a low stool or box.
- **Bending and lifting -** Bend at the knees, not your waist. Keep the load close to the body, lifting with the legs and not the back. If a load is too heavy to handle, ask for help.

Keep stress under control

- **Think positive -** Look for humour in stressful situations.

- **Talk it out** - Share frustrations with your spouse or friends.
- **Relax** - Practise relaxation techniques. Breathe slowly and imagine yourself in a calm place. If your doctor agrees to it try prenatal yoga classes.

Expected weight gain during pregnancy

1st Trimester — 1kg

2nd Trimester — 5kg

3rd Trimester — 5kg

- 11kg is the total weight gain
- In an underweight mother total weight gain can be about 13-14 kgs.
- Total weight gain for an obese mother must not be more than 7kg.

If the mother is expecting twins then ideally the calculated weight gain would differ.

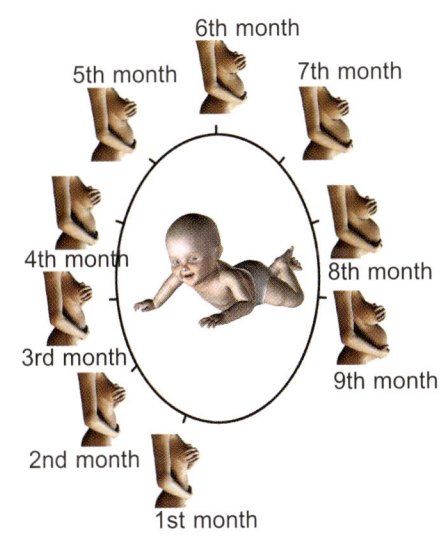

Third Trimester

The seventh month: The foetus now kicks and stretches, and changes position from side to side. The mother is seen to put on weight. Swelling on the feet is often noted. It is better if the feet are propped up off and on during the day.

The eighth month: Daily activities should be continued along with rest at frequent intervals. Heavy lifting or work causing strain should be stopped. By week 32, the foetus's face becomes smooth, and closely resembles that of a newborn. He continues to put on fat. Start preparing the bag for the hospital.

The ninth month: At 36th week the foetus should weigh nearly 6 pounds (2.8 kgs). Weight gain of the foetus is about 1/2 pound (approx.) per week. At around 40 weeks, the foetus is full-term and weighs from 6 to 9 pounds (2.8-3.5 kgs) approximately. The foetus at this stage settles further down into the pelvis. Mother's breathing becomes easier, urination may get frequent. Visit to the doctor will be every week now till the baby is born. By the end of this trimester, the foetus's head will most likely be engaged in the pelvis (more common during first pregnancy). Meanwhile the foetus continues to receive antibodies from the mother through the placenta. Vernix caseosa (a cheesy substance) protects the skin of the foetus from the amniotic fluid. By the end of the pregnancy the mother gains about 11kg (more than her pre-pregnancy weight). Braxton-Hicks Contractions, are common. and are painless. These contractions are usually very irregular, and do not fall into any set pattern, as do real contractions. If the contractions begin to form a regular pattern of 4 or more an hour, be sure to contact the doctor immediately.

Before admission into hospital, get your bag ready.

Your hospital bag should contain :-

- Nighties, toiletries (soap, body wash, talcum, oil, moisturizing lotion, etc)
- Sanitary pads
- Diapers for the baby
- Baby's clothes

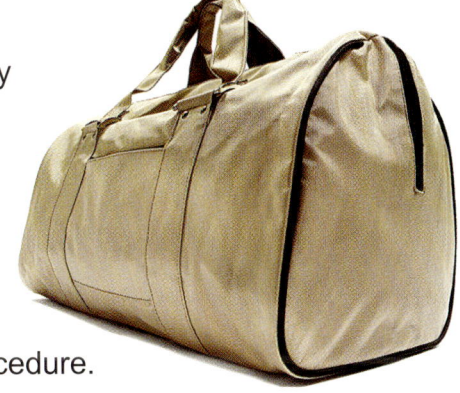

Multiple Pregnancy

A multiple pregnancy is diagnosed with the help of an ultrasound which is done as a routine procedure.

Twins and triplets are multiple pregnancies.

Twins and Their Types

Women over 30 years of age or on fertility drugs are prone to carry more than one foetus. A family history of twins also predisposes the mother to have multiple births. Multiple pregnancy babies have a higher risk of being born prematurely along with higher health risks.

Identical and fraternal twins

Twins are of two basic types – identical and fraternal or non-identical. Identical twins are formed when one fertilised egg splits into two at some time during early pregnancy. Fraternal twins are born when two separate eggs are fertilised by two separate sperms. Identical twins share the same amniotic sac but have separate

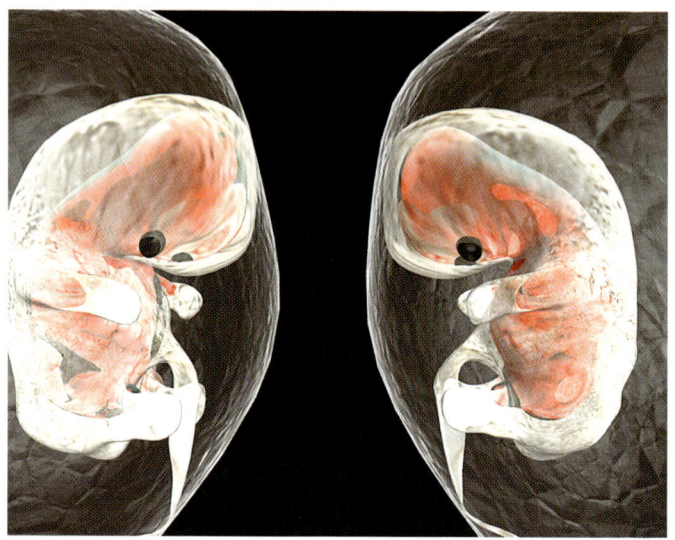

placentas. Fraternal twins usually develop in separate amniotic sacs and have separate placentas.

Siamese or conjoined twins

They are a variation of identical twins. These twins are joined at one or the other body part. Siamese twins, like identical twins look alike and are of the same sex. These twins are joined at some point in their bodies and may also share some organs. They can also be joined from the head, chest, abdomen and hips.

Mirror twins

They are mirror images of each other and are rare. They have organs on the opposite sides. One twin will have the heart on the right side instead of the left and will be opposite-handed to the other twin.

Complications of a multiple pregnancy

- Preterm (or early) labour resulting in premature birth.
- Slow intra-uterine growth restriction of the babies or one twin is due to sharing of all nutrients from the mother
- Birth defects
- Anaemia

Problems during a multiple pregnancy

- Excessive weight gain
- Excessive vomiting
- Gestational diabetes
- Toxaemia of pregnancy (high blood pressure)
- High chances of an operative delivery (Caesarean section)
- Post partum haemorrhage (excessive bleeding after delivery)

When a mother is diagnosed with multiple foetuses she is prescribed more rest than required during a normal pregnancy. Frequent tests should be done to monitor good health of the babies. Dietary modifications may be needed for more nutrition required to meet the mother's needs.

3 Diseases Affecting Mother and Foetus

Irritants During Pregnancy

Some women develop a continuous stuffiness of the nose or nose block during late pregnancy. The presence of certain hormones during this period leads to swelling of mucous membranes inside the nose and sinuses leading to nasal stuffiness. These hormones are actually released for softening the vagina and mouth of the womb in order to ready the womb for the baby's delivery.

Frequency of Urination

Frequent urination during first and third trimester of pregnancy is common.

Five tips to cope with frequent urination: -

- Drink plenty of fluids to keep yourself hydrated during pregnancy.
- Avoid caffeine products like tea, soda or coffee
- Consume most of your fluids during the day to avoid getting up at night frequently to relieve yourself.
- Try and evacuate the bladder completely.

Urine infection –

It should be treated by your doctor. You may need a course of antibiotics, which will not affect your pregnancy. Try passing more urine to flush out infection. Drink plenty of water. You can also have other liquids like barley water, *chaach* (butter milk) light tea, etc.

A healthy mother and a well-cared pregnancy is likely to have fewer complications compared to a mother who has had little prenatal care, a history of chronic disease or a history of complications during pregnancy.

Itching

An itchy skin and redness developing over abdomen, thighs and breasts is due to stretching of the skin. Excessive sweating often aggravates this. Wearing of polyester or any other synthetic fabric can also result in itching. For relief apply Vitamin E oil or Lactocalamine lotion. If itching is not relieved consult your doctor.

Pins and Needles

A feeling of tingling and numbness can be felt in the hands in the morning. This "pin and needles" effect is due to accumulation of fluid on hands and wrists at night.

To relieve this:

- Stretch your hands above your head. Fingers pointing towards the sky, open and close your fists alternatively.
- Reduce the use of oil and salt in your diet.

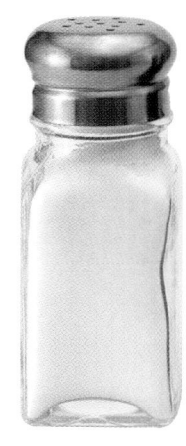
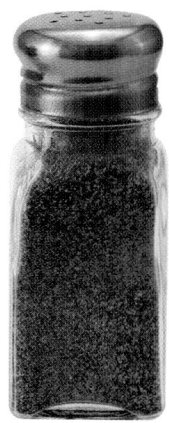

Flatulence or Wind

To avoid excessive flatulence (or wind) avoid rich and spicy food.

Gaseous foods like peas, beans, cabbage, rice and oily food cause flatulence. So try and take less of these.

Nausea, Vomiting and Acidity

The term "morning" sickness arises as it occurs mainly in the morning. It can also be present any time – day or night. To reduce it follow these tips:

- **Avoid triggering of nausea :** Smell of foods at home which are reheated can often make the stomach flip-flop. Avoid anything that seems to trigger nausea.

- **Snack often :** Crackers and other bland foods can be lifesavers when you start to feel nauseated. Keep candy or lemon drops in the mouth. Sipping ginger tea also helps.

- **Drink plenty of fluids :** Drink enough fluids otherwise nausea may get worse. Try sipping water throughout the day.

- **Take it slow in the morning :** Rushing around often contributes to nausea.

- **Get enough sleep :** The more tired you are, the more nauseated you may feel.

Acidity and Indigestion

To avoid acidity, never keep your stomach overfull or empty. Avoid long gaps between meals. Also eat whatever you can digest well like light snacks.

To avoid indigestion or heart burn (acidity) a pregnant woman must:

- Keep a 2 to 3 hour gap between fluid intake and lying down at a slight inclination.
- Have small frequent meals.
- Avoid spicy and oily food.
- Reduce the amount of raw foods in the diet (e.g. apple with skin, excessive salads).

Fatigue

A pregnant woman may feel tired, especially if she is a working lady and cannot take long hours of rest. In that case during the day she should

- Take short, frequent breaks
- Keep an exercise routine
- Go to bed early

Cramps

In the last trimester of pregnancy leg cramps may occur, which can be quite painful. Cramps can be due to :-

- Lack of calcium
- Sluggish circulation
- Low salt (during heat and humidity)
- Lack of Vitamin B and Vitamin E

Remedy

If cramps are experienced at night, try walking on the toes, and then on the heels before bedtime. Also try pressing the outer sides of your feet on the floor. Take a wholesome diet consisting of milk and milk products (cottage cheese, yogurt), green vegetables, whole lentils (dals), salads, fruits and a few nuts.

Constipation and Piles

Women during pregnancy have a tendency to be constipated. This is partly due to wrong eating habits and not drinking enough water.

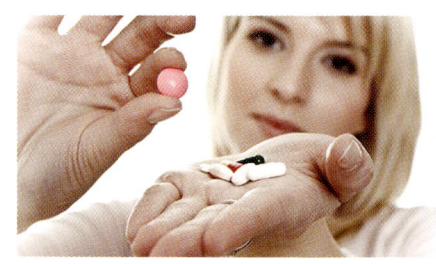

Also, relaxation of muscles of the intestine and pressure of uterus over the rectum causes constipation.

Oral iron intake and inactivity during pregancy is another reason to develop constipation.

During pregnancy constipation and straining to pass stool over a period of time can cause veins around the anus to protrude. This leads to development of piles. To prevent developing piles, avoid spicy and oily food. Consume enough fluids along with fibrous food.

Smoking or Drinking

Women who smoke, chew tobacco or consume alcohol should avoid indulging in these products during pregnancy. In fact, these products should be stopped before a woman gets pregnant. Women who smoke and consume alcohol are often known to have babies with abnormalities.

High Altitude

When women who are used to living in plains visit high altitude, they may develop pregnancy related complications. Hypertension, water retention and an underweight baby are some of the problems one may

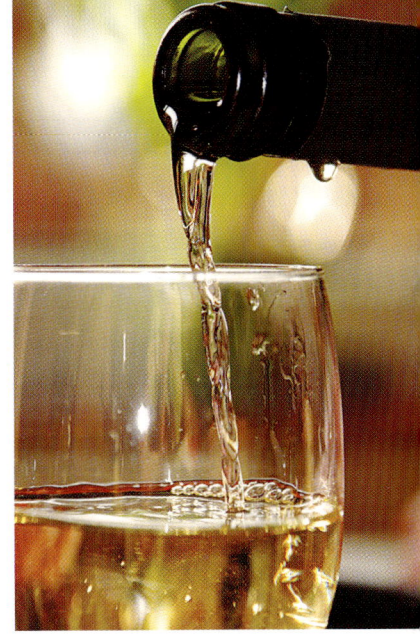

have. High altitude or any other condition depriving the baby of oxygen, e.g. smoking or strenuous exercise should be avoided. A brisk walk should be opted over jogging. Any type of activity the mother participates in should not reach a point of exhaustion.

Extreme Heat

The body overheats easily when you are pregnant. Your body's metabolism at this stage is working overtime. Keep your body cool with the following tips:

- Avoid exercising outside if it is hot.
- Dress lightly and wear airy and light fabrics.
- Even while exercising inside or in an air conditioned room, quit before you overheat yourself and get yourself exhausted.

- If you have been outdoors for a long time, then when you come back home take a shower or bath to become cool.
- Drink plenty of water throughout the day (at least 8 glasses /day)

Controlling the cold

Pregnant mothers do not feel as cold as the normal population. To avoid getting exposed to extreme weather, certain precautions are important. The pregnant mother must dress properly with warm clothes. During winter or windy months the head must be covered with a scarf, cap or hat. Gloves must be worn and legs and feet must be kept warm with proper stockings and socks.

During Pregnancy Keep an Eye on Your

Anaemia

If you are anaemic and pregnant eat nutritious greens. Add mint, coriander *(dhania)*, raisins, dates and other leafy greens in your diet. Remember iron absorption is hindered by tea, coffee and cola. Vitamin C or lime aids absorption of iron.

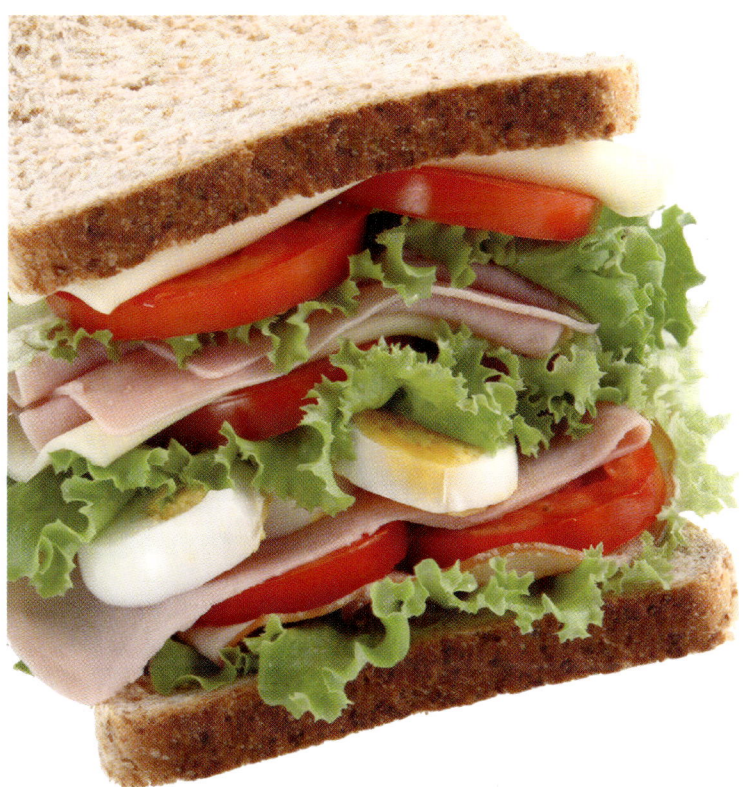

Weight

Excessive weight gain is a result of hunger pangs during pregnancy. Eat before you are hungry. Take three main meals a day and three small snacks. Space them out well, so that you do not get hungry and crave for the wrong kinds of foods. For snacks you can have fruit, sprouts or a bowl of curd. You can also substitute with salad, a brown bread sandwich or a *missi roti*.

Fever

High fever in case of infection (e.g. flu) can affect both mother and the foetus. Do not self medicate, consult your doctor.

Some of the problems which can arise during pregnancy are: -

Preterm labour
When labour starts before the 37th week of pregnancy. The earlier the labour starts the riskier the birth.

Placental problems -
Placenta may cover all or a part of the cervix (*placenta previa*) or the placenta may tear away from the uterine wall too early (placental abruption) or the placenta may grow through the muscles lining of the uterus. This can be diagnosed by ultrasound during pregnancy.

Meconium
Meconium is a thick, sticky green, tar like substance that lines the baby's intestines during pregnancy. This passes out through the baby's anus as stool. If the meconium is present during pregnancy, labour or birth, the foetus should be watched closely for signs of foetal distress.

Foetal Distress
Foetal monitoring is an important function during labour. Foetal distress can be caused by the compression of the cord around the baby's neck, meconium strained liquor or infection in the mother, etc.

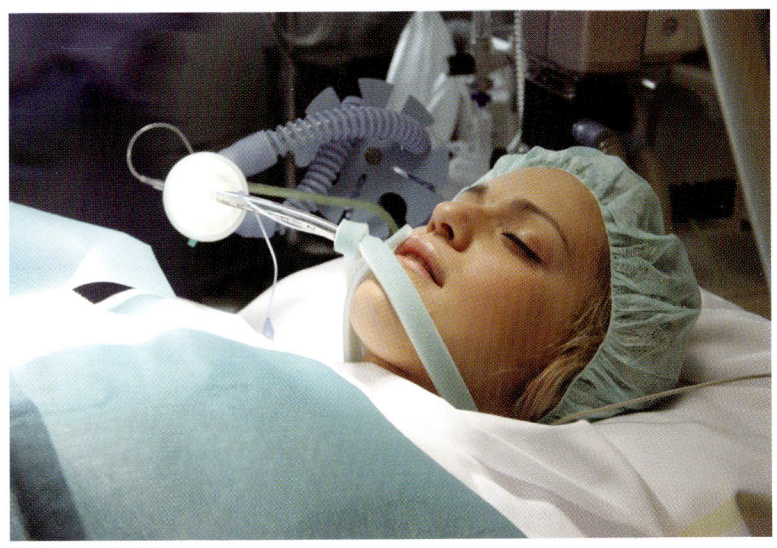

Premature Baby

Premature baby is defined as the baby born between twenty eight and thirty seven weeks of gestation. Premature babies need special care.

Bleeding after delivery

Postpartum Haemorrhage is excessive bleeding after birth.

Some factors which can aggravate it are:

- Multiple gestation (twins, triplets, etc)
- Multigravide – more than 5 previous births
- Induction of labour
- Big baby

Factors which can lead to a Preterm Birth

Factors related to maternal age or disease have shown to increase the risk of preterm birth. They can be one or more of the following :

- Age > 35 yrs
- Age < 18 yrs
- Chromosomal abnormalities
- High blood pressure
- Pre-eclampsia
- Short cervix
- Maternal diabetes
- Any infection e.g present (periodontal, vaginal)
- Twin Pregnancy
- Increased amniotic fluid
- Trauma

Factors relating to a past history of high risk pregnancy also have shown to increase the risk of preterm birth, e.g., vaginal bleeding during labour, prior miscarriage or abortion, multiple pregnancies (twins, triplets), etc.

Ectopic Pregnancy

An ectopic pregnancy is an abnormal pregnancy, which occurs outside the womb, i.e. the uterus. The most common site for an ectopic pregnancy to occur is within one of the fallopian tubes. Normally, it is through the fallopian tube that the egg passes from the ovary to the uterus. In rare cases, ectopic pregnancies can occur in the ovary, stomach area, or cervix. The foetus does not survive during an ectopic pregnancy.

Symptoms of ectopic pregnancy

- Missed periods
- Abnormal vaginal bleeding
- Pain in the lower back or abdomen
- Mild cramping on one side of the pelvis
- Fainting or dizziness, nausea

Your doctor will diagnose ectopic pregnancy based upon the symptoms, signs and the tests conducted on you.

Miscarriage

Consult your doctor for possible signs of miscarriage e.g.:

- When there is severe abdominal pain and it persists for a few hours (even if it is not accompanied by spotting or bleeding)
- Cramps or pain in the lower abdomen persist.
- When there is light spotting for a day or more or if there is heavy bleeding.
- On a previous history of miscarriage any cramps or spotting becomes a case for concern.

Diseases in the mother which can be transmitted to the newborn

Toxoplasmosis –

It is a parasitic infection. Toxoplasmosis is acquired through faeces, raw meat of animals and birds. It is a dormant infection in the human beings. A woman infected by Toxoplasmosis before pregnancy is not affected. It is only when she is pregnant and gets infected that there are 50% chances of passing toxoplasmosis on to the baby.

In the foetus, infection in the brain can result in growth retardation. Once identified Toxoplasmosis can be treated by medication, helping lower the risk to the foetus.

Precautions

for not getting infected with Toxoplasmosis

- Eat cooked eggs and meat (never raw)
- Drink boiled or pasteurized milk.
- Wash fruits and vegetables thoroughly.
- Wash your hands properly before consuming food.
- Protect your food from cockroaches and flies.
- When gardening use gloves.

Rubella

During pregnancy avoid getting exposed to diseases like, rubella, measles, etc If a woman gets measles during the first trimester

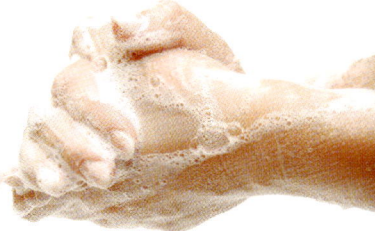

(first three months of pregnancy) the pregnancy would have to be terminated, as the foetus gets affected.

Genital Herpes

It is a cause of great concern. It can present itself with fever, headache, malaise, genital pain, itching on urination and vaginal discharge. The foetus can be affected by this disease. The doctor should be informed if a woman has it. The disease can be transmitted during delivery if the lesions of herpes have blistered and are crusting.

A woman should be careful as to not pass this disease on to her partner. The doctor will prescribe medication for pain and infection. The mother should be guided to take protective steps during pregnancy and delivery. If she is careful the foetus has only about 2-3% chances of getting infected.

Human Immunodeficiency Virus (HIV) and the Pregnant Mother

HIV transmission from mother to child during pregnancy, labour, delivery or breastfeeding is called *perinatal transmission.*

HIV and AIDS

HIV (Human Immunodeficiency Virus) causes AIDS (Acquired Immunodeficiency Syndrome). Taking Anti viral medication can prevent HIV transmission during pregnancy, labour and delivery. If a woman and her partner are HIV positive before she becomes pregnant then pregnancy must be planned and a doctor consulted before the woman decides to conceive. Once deciding to go in for a pregnancy the woman should undergo early intervention through medication, which will help protect her, her partner and her baby. An HIV positive woman with an HIV negative partner can become pregnant by using artificial insemination. This would provide total protection for the man, but HIV transmission to the baby remains. By limiting unprotected sex to the time of ovulation, a couple can reduce the number of opportunities for HIV to be transmitted between them.

The drugs preventing HIV being transmitted from a mother to her baby are called antiretroviral (ARV) drugs.

In developing countries exclusive breast feeding is advised.

Mixed feeding (Breast milk and artificial milk) should be discouraged.

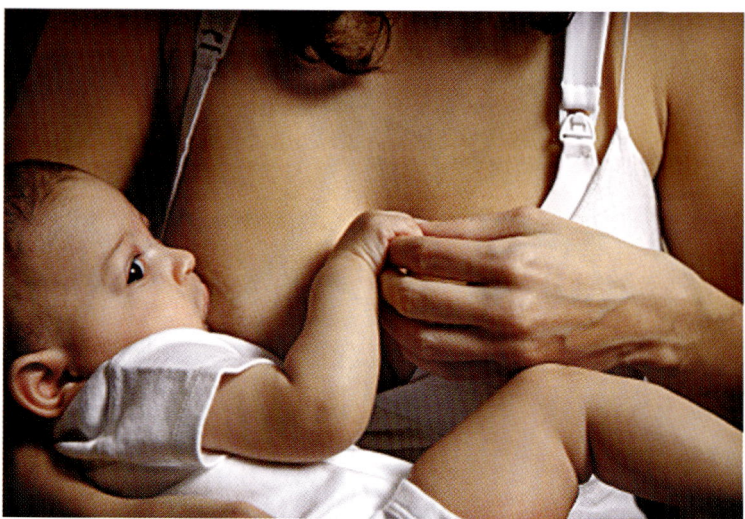

Pregnancy and Fibroids

A fibroid tumour is a mass of compacted muscle and fibrous tissue that grows on the wall or the outside of the uterus.

Symptoms

- Abdominal pain
- Frequent urination
- Constipation
- Back pain or pressure
- Bleeding through vagina

Women between 35 to 45 years of age are more likely to develop larger fibroids.

Causes

Reproductive hormones like estrogen can stimulate cell growth, causing fibroids to form. During pregnancy, the influx of hormones may cause the fibroids to grow in size.

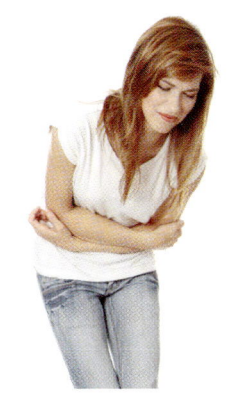

Fibroids usually develop prior to pregnancy. Pregnant women with fibroids may end up having complications. The most common complaint is abdominal pain with light vaginal bleeding. The baby is normally not affected unless the mother has heavy bleeding.

Treatment

Painful fibroids are usually treated with bed rest and medication for pain relief. The symptoms normally subside within a few days.

Pregnancy and Diabetes

Diabetes in a pregnant woman can be:

- Non-insulin dependent diabetes mellitus (NIDDM) or insulin dependent diabetes mellitus (IDDM)
- Gestational diabetes is first recognised during pregnancy

Pregnancy in any woman with a known history of NIDDM must be "Planned"

In a diabetic woman

- Any advised medication to be strictly monitored by the doctor.
- The pregnant woman should be managed on diabetic diet and insulin.
- Glycosylated Haemoglobin level should be well within the "normal" range.
- All NIDDM women planning a pregnancy should be evaluated for the presence of retinopathy and nephropathy.

Management of Diabetes during Pregnancy

- Diet – 35 to 40 calories per kg ideal body weight plus 300 calories. Pregnancy does not require a diet for two.
- If the mother's is blood sugar level is not controlled with diet alone, she will require insulin therapy.
- Blood glucose monitoring by a glucometer should be done three to four times daily and insulin doses adjusted to maintain target levels. Glycosylated haemoglobin estimations should be done every 8 weeks.
- Avoid hypoglycemia
- Antenatal check up of the mother and foetus allows most pregnancies to proceed to full term.

Management During Labour

- Tight control of maternal glycemia is essential throughout labour.

Hypoglycemia in the Newborn

- Neonatal hypoglycemia is defined as blood glucose levels less than 40mg% in full term infants and less than 30 mg% in premature babies.
- An infant of a mother with NIDDM should be checked for blood glucose levels within 30-60 minutes of birth. Checking must be continued at regular intervals till there is no risk of hypoglycemia

Gestational Diabetes

Gestational Diabetes Mellitus is carbohydrate intolerance detected the first time during pregnancy. All pregnant women must undergo testing to rule out gestational diabetes mellitus. GDM screening is usually conducted during 24-28 weeks of pregnancy.

Management of GDM

- Strict calorie restriction is not advisable during pregnancy.
- Blood glucose levels should be assayed at least 2-3 times a week.
- If the fasting blood glucose levels are more than 100mg%, or 2 hour postparandial blood glucose more than 140mg%, the frequency of monitoring should be increased to 2-3 times daily.
- If target values are not met, early initiation of insulin therapy is essential.

Pregnancy and Heart Disease

Is it safe for a woman having heart disease to get pregnant? Yes, depending upon the kind of heart disease she has.

A woman having a history of heart disease, heart murmur, high blood pressure or rheumatic fever should consult with the doctor before she decides to become pregnant.

Once pregnant, the woman needs to be under the care of a cardiologist as well as the obstetrician. Her visits should be at an interval of two weeks till her 28th week of pregnancy. Thereafter her visits should be at weekly intervals or as advised by the doctor.

She should try and keep herself healthy with a balanced diet, adequate rest and not eating out frequently. She should avoid common infections like viral, cold and a bad stomach.

A pregnant woman should avoid exertion. She should report to the hospital in case of breathlessness or extreme fatigue.

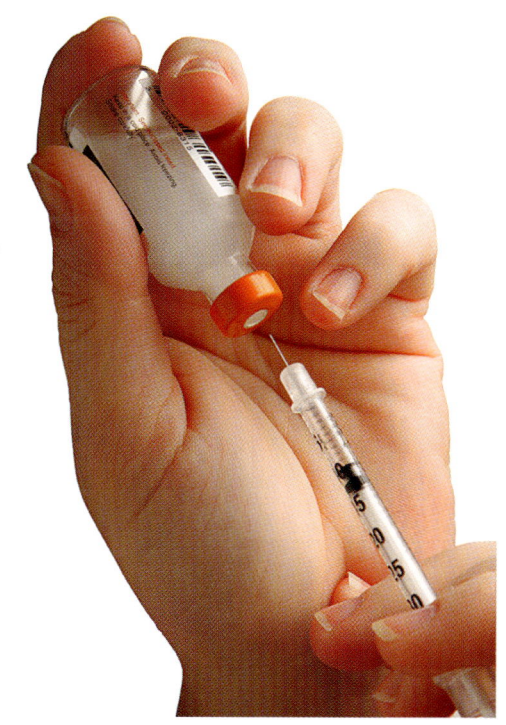

Pregnancy and the Modern Woman

Travel

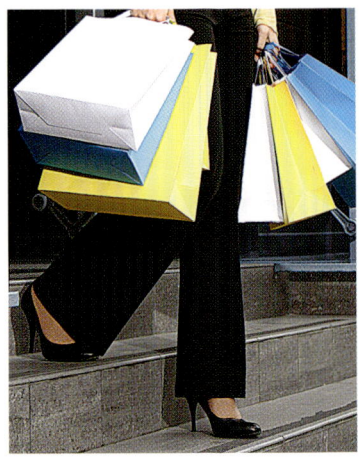

Travelling is not recommended during the early months of pregnancy. Travel by air should be avoided in high risk pregnancy during the first trimester of pregnancy and then during the last 6 weeks of pregnancy. If a miscarriage or bleeding has previously occurred and if a mother is suffering from high blood pressure, then the doctor should be consulted before travelling.

Car Driving

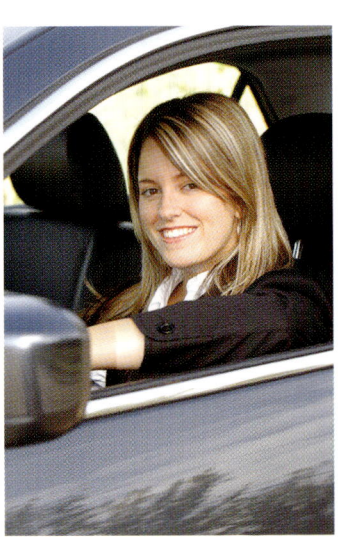

- Avoid driving fast on bumps, speedbrakers and potholes.
- Sudden braking and long hours of travelling should be avoided.
- Drive safely and carefully.
- Comfortable clothes and appropriate shoes should be worn while travelling.

The seat belt should be fastened below the belly and across the pelvis. This would give minimum discomfort to the baby on abrupt breaking as he or she is well cushioned by the amniotic fluid and the uterine muscles (which act as excellent shock absorbers).

Use of Computers or VDU (Visual Display Unit)

It is impossible to prove that the use of VDU in pregnancy is 100 per cent safe. Though a lot of research regarding this aspect has been conducted, evidence of harm to mother or foetus on use of computers has still not been established.

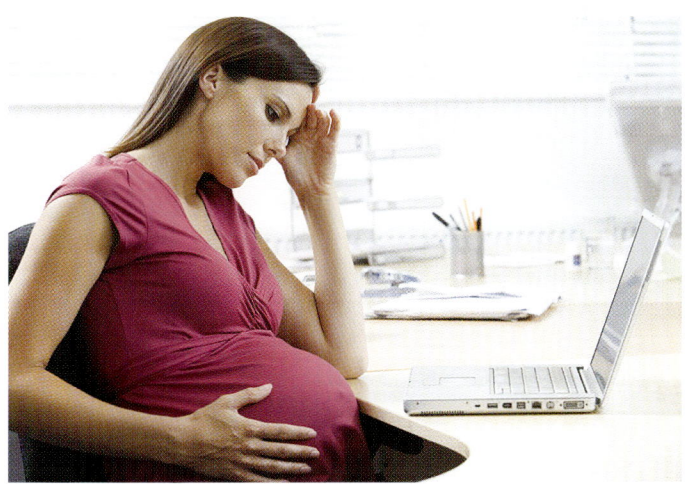

Mobile Phone Usage

Every mobile phone is rated according to the levels of electromagnetic radiation (radio waves) that it emits. This SAR (specific absorption rate) value reflects the maximum amount of energy absorbed by your body when the phone is being used. The higher the phone's SAR, the more radiation is absorbed by the body. The SAR rating is given in your mobile phone instruction manual.

Recommendations made by the International Commission on Non-Ionising Radiation Protection are normally accepted. Non-ionising radiation is unlikely to harm a developing foetus, as it is at the low end of the electromagnetic spectrum.

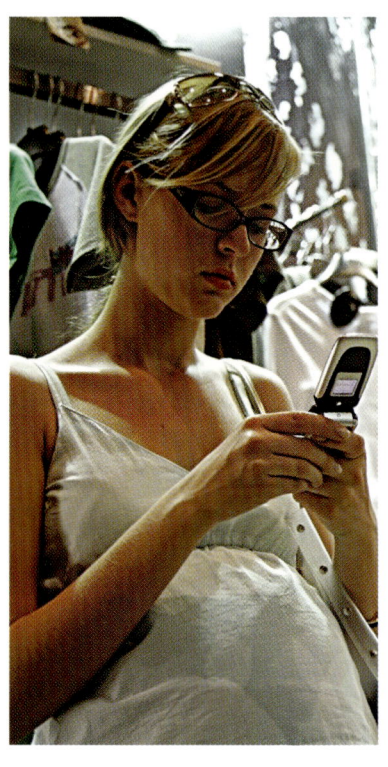

The exposure from the mobile phone can be reduced by:

- Using the phone as little as possible
- Keeping the calls short
- Avoiding use of the phone if the signal strength is low.
- Consider using a hands-free set, to increase the distance between the head and the phone.
- Reading up on the reviews and consumer feedback before buying a phone.

Some Do's and Don'ts During Pregnancy

Do's	Don'ts
(i) Keep the weight within the recommended range.	(i) High heels and uncomfortable footwear should not be worn.
(ii) Sleep on a firm mattress A comfortable position for sleeping along with a body pillow will help in reducing aches and pains.	(ii) Try not to lift abruptly. Very heavy items should not be lifted. Don't lift any item from the floor by bending at your waist. First bend your knees to lift the item.
(iii) Simple exercises like strengthening the abdominal muscles is important.	(iii) Do not sit or stand for a long period of time. Take a little break by walking or stretching.
(iv) Take a nap or stretch back after lunch. Remember, a good nights rest is very important for the mother and foetus. This cannot be substituted by snatching hours of sleep during the day.	(iv) The mother should not overexert herself. The day should be sensibly planned and not too many tasks be listed for the day.
(v) Seasonal vegetables and fruits should be taken. Then body should not be exposed to sudden varying temperatures, as the mother then will be more prone towards infections and allergies.	(v) Avoid too much excitement. A continuous rush is neither good for the mother, nor for the foetus.

4   *Healthy Eating with Safe Exercise During Pregnancy*

The Daily Balanced Diet

During pregnancy a woman's diet should consist of:

- 4-5 helpings of whole grain and complex carbohydrates
- 2-3 helpings of foods with first class proteins.
- 3 helpings of green, leafy and yellow vegetables or fruits
- 4 helpings of foods rich in calcium (4 helpings during pregnancy, and 5 helpings during lactation)
- 2 helpings of food rich in vitamin C
- 2 helpings of food rich in iron
- 8-10 glasses of water
- Supplements of folic acid, calcium and iron to be taken according to the doctor's recommendation.

Pregnancy and Nutrition

Nutrients are delivered from the mother to the child via the placenta. Do not eat less than 2400 calories per day. Pregnant women should increase their calorific intake by at least 300 calories per day.

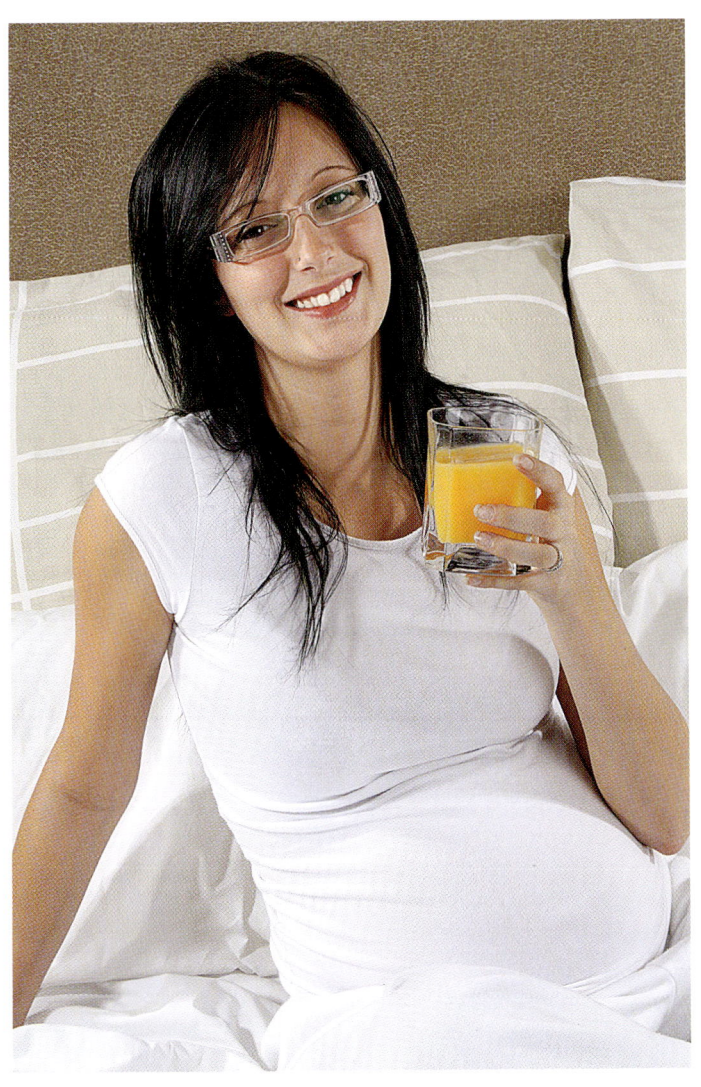

Vitamins and Minerals Required During Pregnancy

Fat Soluble

- **Vitamin A** - Vital for cellular differentiation and foetal development

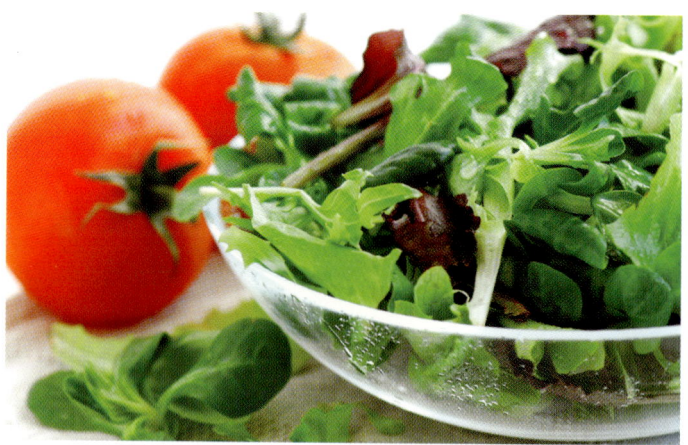

- **Vitamin D** - Vital for foetal skeletal development and calcium absorption. There should be regular exposure to the sun. Vitamin D fortified milk is recommended
- **Vitamin E**
- **Vitamin K**

Water Soluble

- **Vitamin C** - Additional requirement is about 10 mg per day during pregnancy.
- **Thiamine** - Approximately 0.4 mg per day of additional requirement. Insufficient intake can

cause foetal heart abnormalities and muscle weakness
- **Vitamin B 6** - Important for amino acid (protein) metabolism. 0.6 mg per day of additional requirement.
- **Niacin** - Additional 2 mg per day requirement
- **Folic acid (Folate) -** Insufficient intake may result in anemia during pregnancy. Folate deficiency may increase risk of birth defects (neural and cardiac defects) and impair foetal growth. Recommended intake is 400 mcg per day.
- **Vitamin B 12** - Recommended intake is approximately 2.0 mcg per day.

Minerals/ Trace Elements (approximately)

- **Calcium** – RDA Recommended Dietary Advice) during pregnancy is 1200 mg.
- **Magnesium** - RDA during pregnancy is 320 mg.
- **Iodine** – Its deficiency can cause thyroid abnormalities in both the mother and the foetus
- **Iron** - Deficiency may cause low birth weight, pre-term birth, and perinatal mortality. Intake of iron during pregnancy should be approximately 40 mg. As normal diets often fall short on iron intake, a supplement is mostly recommended.
- **Zinc** - Deficiency may result in an increased risk of pregnancy complications and birth defects. RDA during pregnancy is 15 mg.

- **Water** - It is recommended that pregnant women consume at least 2.5 litres of fluids per day.

Potentially Harmful Substances during Pregnancy

- **Smoking** – It can increase the risk of preterm delivery, perinatal mortality or spontaneous abortion.
- **Caffeine** – Taking too much of caffeine can cause abortion, inhibit foetal growth, cause retardation and or inhibit calcium and iron absorption.
- **Alcohol** –Intake of alcohol during pregnancy can cause prenatal and/ or postnatal growth retardation, nervous system abnormalities and intellectual impairment. It can also lead to cardiac or genital abnormalities.

Healthy nutrition is basic for both mother and foetus. The mother can be a vegetarian or non-vegetarian. Many mothers like only vegetarian food during pregnancy, others crave for non-vegetarian nibbles. The advice is to eat what the body demands, keeping in mind its nutritious value.

Source of Nutrition	Foods
Proteins	Milk, yogurt, paneer, cheese, tofu, peas, all kinds of beans and dals, all kinds of nuts, poultry, lamb, pork, beef, kidneys, all kinds of fish and eggs.
Carbohydrates	Sugar, breads, cereals, rice, potatoes, pastas

Fats	Milk, cream, cheese, butter, margarine, cooking oil, cooking fats, mayonnaise, salad dressings, and nuts, bacon, lard.
Vitamin A	Fish oils, egg yolk, milk, cheese, butter, margarine, fruits like bananas, peaches and apricots, carrots, brussel sprouts, spinach, tomatoes, turnips, beetroots.
Vitamin B1	Beans, peas, all kinds of nuts, wheat, unpolished rice, soya bean, yeast, eggs, liver, kidneys, brain, heart, seafoods and fish oils.
Vitamin B2	Meats like liver, kidneys, heart, brain. All kinds of fish, nuts, milk, cheese, cream, whole wheat, peas and beans.
Vitamin C	All citrus fruits like oranges, grapefruit, melons, strawberries and black currants. Vegetables like tomatoes, cabbage, lettuce, carrots, radish, brussel sprouts, and broccoli. Remember Vitamin C gets destroyed on cooking or heating.
Vitamin D	Fish oils and fish extracts. Animal fats and eggs. Milk and milk products like cheese and butter.

Source of Nutrition	Foods
Vitamin E	Wheat germ oil. Vitamin E is also present in limited amounts in eggs, milk, butter, cheese, unpolished rice, whole wheat bread and wheat.
Other nutrients and minerals	
Iron	Non-vegetarian: meats, especially liver and kidneys. Vegetarian: eggs, spinach, cabbage, brussel sprouts and broccoli.
Calcium	Milk and milk products, e.g. cheese, butter, etc. Also protein in spinach, broccoli, nuts, eggs, and fish.
Folic Acid	Green leafy vegetables, liver and kidneys.
Phosphorus	Seafoods, cheese, eggs, milk, meat, onions and whole wheat bread.
Copper Iodine	Meat, liver, cheese and beans. Iodine is present in all fish foods, fish extracts and Iodised salt.
Manganese	Wheat products, green vegetables, beans, peas. Fruits: Apple, bananas, raspberries, pears, papaya, pineapple, peaches, apricots, mango. Vegetables: Broccoli, turnip, carrots, lettuce, spinach, sweet potatoes, parsley, ladies' fingers, mushrooms, asparagus, potatoes.

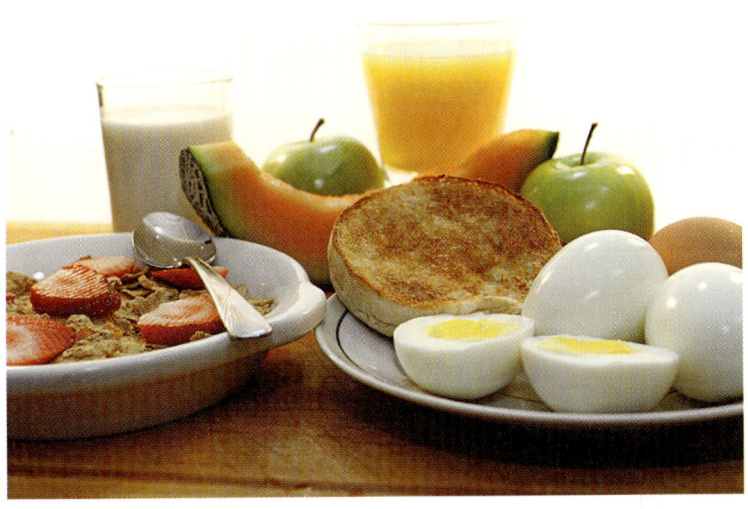

Dietary Supplements

Vitamins, iron and calcium are essential in the diet. Lack of folic acid in the first trimester is shown to increase the risk of neural tube defects, lip and palate deformities in the foetus. Most doctors also recommend daily supplements of folic acid starting from the first month and iron and calcium after the first trimester. Specially iron-fortified multivitamin supplements formulated for pregnancy and lactation are also available. Although most supplements are available over the counter, make sure that the mother consults the doctor regarding their usage.

Tips Supporting Healthy Eating

- **Calories** – Remember if you have an average weight you need additional 300 cals/day only. It is unwise to consume more calories than required. Consume calories which are nutritious, e.g. whole wheat, bread and fruits. Avoid empty calories like sugar and sugary products

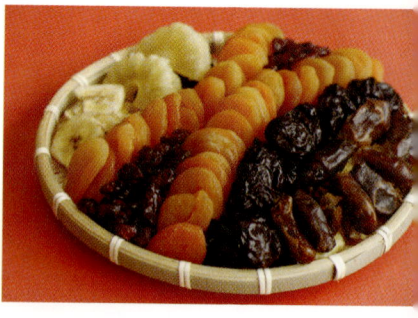

- **Carbohydrates** – The complex ones (cereals, fresh fruits, vegetables, whole grain bread, hot potatoes with skin) are rich in essential vitamins, minerals and fibres. Eating lots of fibre can help reduce the risk of developing gestational diabetes.

- **Sugar** – For the sugary taste consume fruits or fruit juices. Dried apricots, dates, raisins, etc. can be taken as a sweet. Along with the sweetness, these fruits are rich in vitamins and phytochemicals (chemicals defending against ageing and disease)

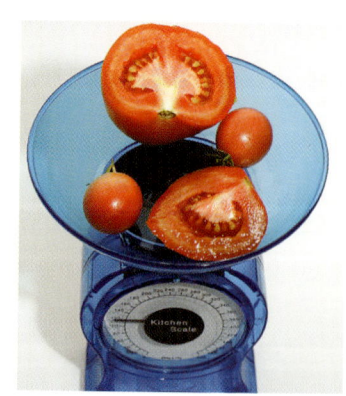

- **Protein rich foods** – They have to be chosen wisely. 60-70 gms of protein, divided into three meals can be taken each day. Keep the fat content in the proteins low. Whole grain along with low fat cheese and lean meats like turkey, etc. can be taken.

- **No starving** – The foetus growing in your body needs regular nourishment. Even if you are not feeling hungry the foetus needs to be nourished. Don't skip meals. Regular meals and two snacks are best for a well-nourished mother and foetus.

Sex During Pregnancy

Though sex is considered safe during normal pregnancy, it is better to avoid sex during the first 6 weeks and last six week of pregnancy. Normal pregnancy is defined as one which is at low risk for complications or any medical disorder. Many expectant mothers find that their desire for sex fluctuates. Some also find sex becoming uncomfortable as their body grows. One should not have sex with a partner whose sexual history is unknown. Sex also should be avoided with one who may have sexually transmitted diseases like herpes, HIV, etc.

Sexual intercourse is not advised when the following risk factors are present:

- A history or threat of miscarriage
- A history of preterm labour
- Unexplained vaginal bleeding, discharge, or cramping.
- Amniotic fluid leakage
- Placenta praevia (here the placenta – the blood-rich structure that nourishes the foetus is situated so low that it covers the cervix).
- Incompetent cervix (here the cervix is weakened and it dilates) opens prematurely, raising the risk for miscarriage or premature delivery.
- If the mother is carrying twins, triplets, etc.

Sex and the baby

The foetus is fully protected by the amniotic sac (The thin-walled bag that holds the foetus and surrounding fluid) and the strong muscles of the uterus. A thick mucus plug seals the cervix and helps guard against infection. The penis does not come into contact with the foetus during sex.

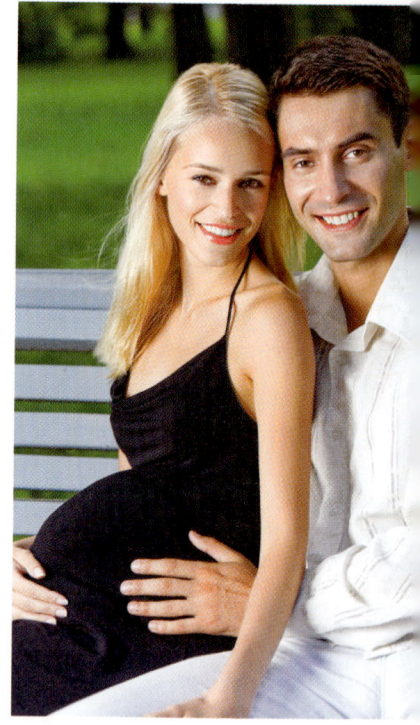

Intercourse and contractions

Semen contains a chemical that stimulates contractions. In cases of high risk pregnancies doctors do not advise sex, especially during the first trimester and during the last weeks of pregnancy.

Exercise and Pregnancy

Exercising releases endorphins (naturally occurring chemicals in your brain). These chemicals make the mother feel better. Exercising helps : -

- Relieve backaches and improve the posture by strengthening and toning the muscles (especially the back, butt, and thighs)
- Prevents wear and tear of the joints (which become loose during pregnancy due to normal hormonal changes)

- Prevents constipation
- Helps the pregnant woman to sleep better, relieving stress and anxiety.
- Prepares the body for delivery. Strong muscles and a fit heart help in easier birth of the baby.
- Exercise during pregnancy helps the mother gain less fat and weight. The mother should not try to lose weight by exercising during pregnancy.

Safe Exercising During Pregnancy

If the mother had exercised regularly before becoming pregnant, the program should be continued. The exercises should be modified as required. If a lady was not fit before she became pregnant, she should begin slowly and build up gradually.

If there are any concerns regarding exercise, discuss it with your doctor. Your exercise may be curtailed or stopped during:

- Pregnancy-induced high blood pressure
- Early uterine contractions
- Vaginal bleeding
- Premature rupture of the membranes (known as the water, i.e. the fluid in the amniotic sac around the foetus breaking early)

Exercises to do during Pregnancy

- During pregnancy, you can swim, do water aerobics, yoga, pilates, biking, or walking.

- A combination of cardio (aerobic), strength, and flexibility exercises can also be done.
- The best exercise for an expecting mother is walking. Start with a moderately brisk pace for a mile. Add a couple of minutes every week and slowly pick up the pace. First 5 minutes are kept to warm up and use the last 5 minutes to cool down.

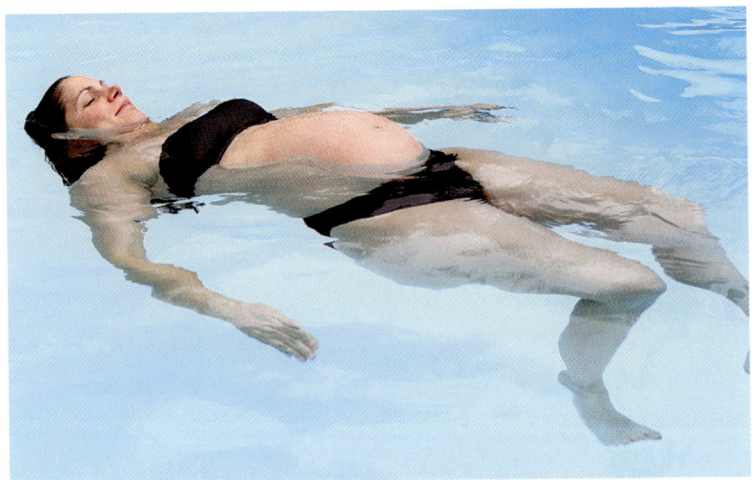

Whatever type of exercise is decided upon must suit the mother and the foetus. Energy level at this stage may also vary greatly from day-to-day. As the foetus grows, there is decreased ability to breathe in more air.

The signs of lack of oxygenation can be:

- Fatigue
- Dizziness
- Shortness of breath

- Heart palpitations (your heart pounding in your chest)

Exercises to Avoid

- After the first trimester of pregnancy, exercises requiring the mother to lie flat on the abdomen should be avoided.
- Any activity requiring leaping, a sudden change of direction can risk abdominal injury and should be avoided.
- Aerobics and workouts also have to be conducted carefully.
- Getting exhausted on exercising should be avoided.

On exercising consult the doctor if there is: -

- Vaginal bleeding
- Unusual pain
- Dizziness or lightheadedness
- Unusual shortness of breath
- Racing heartbeat or chest pain
- Uterine contractions
- Fluid leaking from the vagina

Kegel Exercises

Kegel exercises are often used to reduce incontinence (the leakage of urine) caused by the weight of the baby on their bladder. Kegels help to strengthen the 'pelvic floor muscles' (these muscles aid in urination control).

Squeeze these muscles for a few seconds, and then relax. The abdominal muscles should not be involved.

When performing Kegel exercises:

- Don't tighten other muscles (stomach or legs) at the same time.
- Breath should not be held while you exercise. It is important that the body and muscles continue to receive oxygen while any type of exercise is performed.

While exercising!

- Dress comfortably in loose-fitting clothes and wear a supportive bra to protect your breasts.
- Even 5 minutes a day is a good start if the mother has been inactive. Add 5 minutes each week until 30 minutes are reached.
- Drink plenty of water to avoid overheating and dehydration.
- Skip exercises, if unwell.
- On hot, humid days. Opt for a walk in a room or in an air-conditioned mall.

5   Later Half of Pregnancy and the "D Day"

Later Half of Pregnancy

A few problems can arise in the later half of pregnancy. Proper care and regular check ups can ease these hiccups and not cause serious trouble.

Swollen Ankles and Feet

Swollen ankles and feet are actually edema, i.e. excess fluid collecting in your tissues. The swelling during pregnancy is because of retention of more water. This results in some fluid shifting into the tissues. The enlarging uterus also puts pressure on the pelvic veins and vena cava (the large vein on the right side of the body that carries blood from the lower limbs back to the heart). This increased pressure slows the return of blood from the legs upwards leading to the pool. This in turn forces fluid from the veins into the feet and ankle tissues. Edema is seen during the third trimester of pregnancy especially at the end of the day.

A certain amount of edema on the ankles is normal in the ankles and feet during pregnancy, which should get relieved on rest. Some mild swelling in your hands may also develop. If swelling on the face or puffiness around your eyes is seen or rings get tight on your fingers, consult your doctor. You may be developing pre-eclampsia.

Pre-eclampsia

Pre-eclampsia is known as toxemia of pregnancy-induced hypertension. It is a condition which presents with high blood pressure, fluid retention and protein in urine which is seen in the second half of pregnancy. It can be either mild or severe. In severe cases it can restrict blood flow to the placenta and could seriously harm the foetus.

Women at risk of pre-eclampsia:

- A first-time mother
- Women carrying twins, triplets, teenage mothers and women older than 40 years of age.
- Women who have had high blood pressure or kidney disease prior to pregnancy.
- Women whose sisters and mothers had pre-eclampsia.

To detect pre-eclampsia

At each prenatal checkup the doctor or the healthcare provider will check the blood pressure, urine albumin levels along with any other blood tests required.

Symptoms of pre-eclampsia

- If, after the 20th week of pregnancy, the blood pressure of the mother rises to 140/90 or more (especially if she never had high blood pressure earlier) on two occasions (6 hours apart).

- Sudden weight gain unrelated to excess food intake
- Severe swelling of the hands, feet and face
- Unexplained headaches
- Vision disturbances, e.g. blurred vision
- Protein in the urine or very low urine output

Pre-eclampsia and the baby

Pre-eclampsia prevents the placenta from getting enough blood. If the placenta does not get enough blood, the foetus gets less oxygen and nutrition. This can result in low birth weight / IUGR (intra uterine growth restriction)

Prevention:

- Increased bed rest
- Do not use extra salt in your meals.
- Monitor your blood pressure.
- Drink 6-8 glasses of water a day.
- Avoid fried and junk food.
- Elevate your feet several times during the day.
- Avoid drinking alcohol or caffeinated products.

Medication if required may be suggested by your doctor.

Treatment

If a patient is attending regular antenatal checkups, symptoms of pre-eclampsia are detected early.

Management

The ultimate treatment however is delivery. That is the only cure for a pregnant woman. The condition of the foetus should be assessed regularly during pregnancy.

High Risk Pregnancy

In a high risk pregnancy the mother or the developing foetus or both are at higher than normal risk for complications. This can be during pregnancy and or post birth.

Certain factors responsible for high risk pregnancy

- Age : less than 15 years or older than 35 years
- Overweight or underweight
- Problems during previous pregnancies
- Pre-existing health conditions, e.g. high blood pressure, diabetes, HIV

Advice

- Rest as much as possible.
- The mother should put up her feet whenever possible and place them on a stool at work or on the bed if at home. Crossing of legs while sitting to be avoided.
- The legs should be stretched frequently while sitting. Ankles should be rotated and the toes wiggled. Regular breaks from sitting or standing should be taken. This helps the blood circulating in the body.
- Comfortable shoes should be worn to accommodate the swelling.
- Socks or stockings which have tight bands around the ankles or calves should not be worn.

- Plenty of water should be taken.
- Doctor's advice on medication and rest should be followed.
- Exercise regularly especially walking and swimming.
- Preserved, junk or highly salted foods should be avoided.
- The increased pressure can be relieved on the veins by lying on the side. Lying down on left side works best as the vena cava is on the right side of the body.

On the D-day

A normal delivery is a healthy option for mother and child. In case it has been decided otherwise, the decision for any other delivery mode is best taken by the obstetrician.

Presentation, position and the baby

Normally the head of the baby is set near the pelvis around eighth month of pregnancy. It is the head-down position. If the presentation is head first, the heartbeat of the baby is heard at the lower half of the abdomen.

In the case of a breech presentation, the foetus will have its bottom or feet having descended in the pelvis.

Frank breech – legs are folded up against the face

Footling presentation – foot of the foetus is pointing downwards.

Transverse position – occurs when the foetus lies sideways in the uterus.

Caesarean Section

If due to a number of reasons a baby cannot be delivered normally, a surgical extraction is done from the womb. Caesarean childbirth is a surgery conducted to deliver a baby through an incision in the abdomen.

They can be various Indications for Caesarean Section.

- The doctor will advise the mother if it is needed.

Other Types of Delivery

- **Forceps delivery:** – It is to aid the birth of the baby. Forceps are used if the mother is suffering from certain diseases, e.g. high blood pressure, heart disease. It is also used if the mother is unable to push the baby out of the passage.
- **Vaccum delivery** – It is another mode to help the birth of the baby.

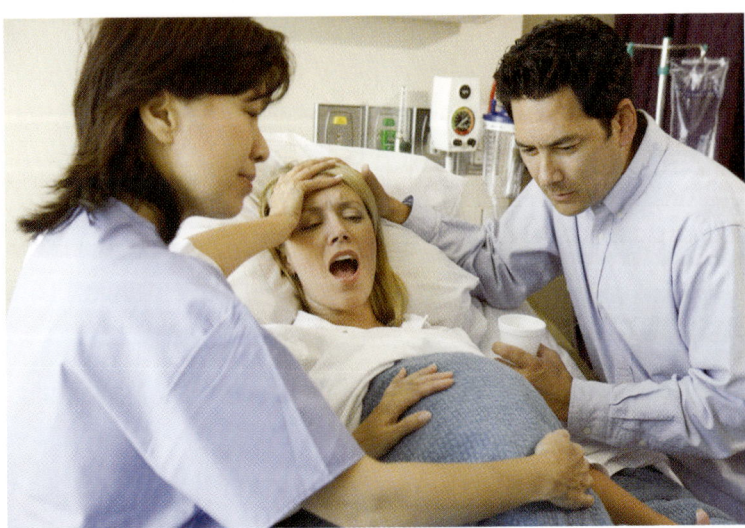

Patient Controlled Epidural Analgesia (PCEA)

A mother being helped to deliver normally can be given PCEA. PCEA provides excellent pain relief. It also provides several advantages including the ability to minimize drug dosage, flexibility and benefits of self administration. This technique is of great benefit since self control and maintenance of self esteem are vital to a positive experience during child birth.

Relief of labour pain is through epidural block. In an epidural block, pain-relieving medicines are injected in the mother's lower back. A small tubing is inserted into this space through a needle. The needle is removed and a catheter is fixed for injecting drugs. This makes it possible to repeat the medication or give it continuously through the catheter. PCEA does not affect the baby and the baby remains active.

The uterine contractions remain normal. The mother remains aware of the contractions as they are painless and help in delivery of the baby by pushing as in a normal delivery. Delivery time may get prolonged. This type of pain relief is also not addictive.

At the end of the labour, when the baby is born, the mother's nine months of pregnancy are behind. Her safe and healthy pregnancy has brought good results. The birth of a child is a moment never forgotten. The mother now looks forward to holding and feeding the baby. The relief and joy says it all.

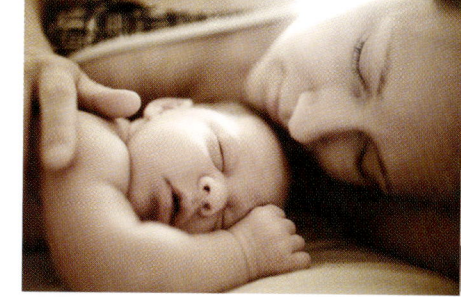

Myths and Fact File

Myth – A pregnant women should eat double, both for herself and her unborn baby.

Fact – A nutritious and balanced diet (carbohydrates, fats, vitamins and minerals + 300 more calories) and 60gm protein are required normally for both the foetus and the mother. A pregnant woman does not need to eat double.

Myth – During pregnancy, a woman should take lot of rest and not work much.

Fact – Unless recommended otherwise by the doctor, a pregnant woman must lead a normal life. A certain amount of exercise, daily work routine and some amount of rest is all that is required for a healthy pregnancy.

Myth – Pregnancy should be terminated if the mother is on anti-tubercular drugs.

Fact – For a pregnant woman with tuberculosis pregnancy need not to be terminated. Under her doctors close supervision, the woman should continue her pregnancy, childbirth and breastfeeding. It is only in active tuberculosis that the baby after delivery is kept away from the mother.

Myth – Smoking does not affect the baby.

Fact – Women who smoke are known to have low weight babies and an increased risk of still birth. In fact, a woman should stop smoking, when she plans to get pregnant.